ULCERATIVE COLITIS DIET COOKBOOK

Delicious Recipes For Inflammatory Bowel Disease Management, Easy Meals For Digestive Health, And Nutritional Healing

DR ELIAN GRIFFIN

Copyright © [Elian Griffin] [2024]. All rights reserved.

Without the publisher's prior written consent, no portion of this publication may be copied, distributed, or transmitted in any way, including by photocopying, recording, or other mechanical or electronic means, with the exception of brief quotations used in all critical reviews.

DISCLAIMER

The nutritional recommendations and recipes in this book are meant solely for informative reasons. They are not meant to replace the counsel, diagnosis, or care of a qualified medical expert. If you have any doubts about a medical condition or dietary requirements, you should always see your physician or another trained healthcare expert.

All reasonable efforts have been taken by the author and publisher to ensure that the information contained in this book is correct as of the date of publication. Recommendations may alter, though, as medical knowledge is always changing. When using any of the recipes or instructions found here, the user assumes all liability and assumes no risk, whether personal or otherwise. People who have certain dietary requirements or medical issues should speak with a healthcare provider for personalized guidance. The given recipes are only ideas; you may need to adjust them to suit your own nutritional needs, tastes, and tolerances.

When you use this book, you agree to release the publisher, the author, and their representatives from any liability for any claims, damages, liabilities, costs, or expenditures resulting from your use of the book.

TABLE OF CONTENTS

CHAPTER ONE 15
ULCERATIVE COLITIS DIET INTRODUCTION 15
- DEFINITION AND SYNOPSIS 15
- SIGNS AND PROGNOSIS 16
- REASONS AND DANGER ELEMENTS 17
- EFFECTS ON DAY-TO-DAY LIVING 18
- DIET IS IMPORTANT FOR MANAGEMENT 19

CHAPTER TWO 21
DIETARY INTERVENTIONS FOR ULCERATIVE COLITIS 21
- THE IMPACT OF FOOD ON INFLAMMATION 21
- RECOGNIZING FOOD TRIGGERS 22
- ADVANTAGES OF A CUSTOMIZED DIET PLAN 24
- UC PATIENTS' NUTRITIONAL REQUIREMENTS 25
- TYPICAL DIETARY STRATEGIES 27

CHAPTER THREE 29
CRUCIAL ELEMENTS FOR INFLAMMATORY BOWEL DISEASE 29
- FIBER'S SIGNIFICANCE 29
- PROBIOTICS AND PREBIOTICS' ROLES 30
- MINERALS AND VITAMINS TO PAY ATTENTION TO 32
- HYDRATION: ITS ADVANTAGES 33
- SUPPLEMENTS FOR EXTRA ASSISTANCE 35

CHAPTER FOUR 37
CREATING A DIET PLAN FOR ULCERATIVE COLITIS 37
- CREATING DIETARY OBJECTIVES 37

MAKING A WELL-COMPOSED MEAL PLAN	39
TIPS FOR GROCERY SHOPPING	40
EXAMINING NUTRITION LABELS	42
ORGANIZING MEALS FOR CONVENIENCE	43
CHAPTER FIVE	**45**
GETTING STARTED	45
FUNDAMENTAL COOKING METHODS	45
ESSENTIAL KITCHEN ITEMS FOR UC-FRIENDLY COOKING	46
SAFE FOOD HANDLING PROCEDURES	48
ADVICE ON HOW TO LOWER FOOD CONTAMINATION	49
MODIFYING RECIPES TO MAKE MEALS UC-FRIENDLY	50
CHAPTER SIX	**53**
MEAL PLANNING AND PREPARATION	53
COMPREHENDING MACRONUTRIENTS	53
PROTEIN, CARBOHYDRATE, AND FAT EQUILIBRIUM	54
FIBER'S SIGNIFICANCE AND HOW TO INCLUDE IT	55
EXAMPLE MEAL SCHEDULES FOR VARIOUS UC STAGES	57
CHANGING MEAL PLANS IN RESPONSE TO SYMPTOMS	58
RECIPES FOR BREAKFAST	60
SMOOTHIES TO PROMOTE DIGESTIVE HEALTH	60
SIMPLE-TO-DIGEST OATMEAL RECIPES	61
HIGH-PROTEIN EGG RECIPES	62
WAFFLES & PANCAKES THAT ARE UC-FRIENDLY	64
OPTIONS FOR DAIRY-FREE YOGURT	65
RECIPES FOR LUNCH	67

- SIMPLE AND LIGHT SALADS 67
- HEALTHY BROTHS & SOUPS 68
- SANDWICHES AND WRAPS WITH LEAN PROTEIN 69
- EASY GRAIN BOWLS 70
- SIDE DISHES MADE WITH VEGETABLES 71

RECIPES FOR DINNER 72
- PASTA DISHES THAT ARE UC-FRIENDLY 72
- RICH STEWS AND CASSEROLES 72
- OPTIONS FOR GRILLED AND BAKED FISH 73
- VEGETARIAN DINNER IDEAS 74
- COMFORT FOOD FOR FLARE-UPS 75

RECIPES FOR SNACKS AND APPETIZERS 76
- SNACKS GOOD FOR THE STOMACH 76
- SIMPLE-TO-PROCESS APPETIZERS 77
- IDEAS FOR PROBIOTIC-RICH SNACKS 78
- FAST AND WHOLESOME DIPS 79
- ON-THE-GO PORTABLE SNACKS 80

DESSERT RECIPES 81
- SUGAR-FREE DESSERT SELECTIONS 81
- FRUIT-BASED SWEETS 82
- NON-DAIRY ICE CREAMS 83
- GUT-RELEASING GELATIN TREATS 84
- UC-FRIENDLY PASTRIES 84

DRINKS AND SMOOTHIES 86
- DRINKS THAT REHYDRATE FOR UC 86

    TEAS WITH ANTI-INFLAMMATION 87

    SMOOTHIES PACKED WITH NUTRIENTS 89

    MAKE YOUR ELECTROLYTE DRINKS 90

    DRINKING AND UC: THINGS TO CONSIDER 91

CHAPTER SEVEN 93

    FREQUENTLY ASKED QUESTIONS 93

        HANDLING RELAPSES AND DIETARY MODIFICATIONS 93

        HANDLING MALNUTRITION AND WEIGHT LOSS 94

        UC TRAVELING AND DINING OUT 95

        FOOD ALLERGIES AND SENSITIVITIES 96

        LONG-TERM DIETARY MANAGEMENT STRATEGIES 97

ABOUT THE BOOK

The "Ulcerative Colitis Diet Cookbook" is an essential tool for anyone attempting to manage ulcerative colitis (UC) through dietary decisions. It starts with an in-depth introduction to ulcerative colitis, which includes a definition, summary, and explanation of the illness, its symptoms, and diagnostic techniques. It then explores the causes and risk factors of UC and talks about the major effects this chronic condition can have on day-to-day living. Stressing the critical role that diet plays in managing UC, the book lays the groundwork for understanding how particular dietary strategies can help control inflammation and enhance quality of life.

Examining how food affects the body's inflammatory levels and identifying common trigger foods that can worsen symptoms; the book explores the role of diet in managing ulcerative colitis. It emphasizes the advantages of a customized diet plan, making sure readers are aware of the nutritional requirements unique to UC patients.

It also covers common dietary approaches, giving readers a starting point for creating a customized and successful eating plan.

Essential nutrients are critical to the management of ulcerative colitis (UC), and this cookbook describes the role of fiber, probiotics, and probiotics in preserving gut health; it lists the vitamins and minerals that are especially helpful for UC patients; it stresses the importance of staying hydrated; and it covers the role of supplements in offering supplemental nutritional support so that readers are fully informed about their dietary requirements.

The book provides helpful advice on setting dietary goals, creating balanced meal plans, and grocery shopping tips that cater to the needs of those with ulcerative colitis. It also includes meal prep and label reading tips, which make it easier for readers to maintain a healthy diet even with a busy lifestyle. Planning an ulcerative colitis-friendly diet requires careful consideration and strategic planning.

Recipes are adapted to be UC-friendly, ensuring that meals are both delicious and suitable for managing the condition. Cooking with UC in mind involves specific techniques and practices, and this book provides a detailed guide to basic cooking techniques that are suitable for UC patients. It lists kitchen essentials for UC-friendly cooking and offers tips for safe food handling and reducing food contamination.

A well-balanced meal plan is essential, and the book walks readers through the significance of fiber, the importance of understanding macronutrients, and how to balance protein, carbs, and fats. It also includes sample meal plans that are customized for various stages of UC and offer guidance on modifying meal plans in response to symptoms, allowing readers to remain adaptable and in tune with their bodies.

There is a wide range of recipes for breakfast, lunch, dinner, snacks, and desserts that are all made to be easy on the digestive tract and still taste good. Breakfast options include protein-rich egg dishes, gut-health smoothies, easy-to-digest oatmeal variations, lean protein wraps and sandwiches, light and easy salads, nourishing soups and broths, simple grain bowls, and vegetable-based side dishes. Dinner options include UC-friendly pasta dishes, hearty stews and casseroles, grilled and baked fish options, vegetarian dinner ideas, and comfort food for flare-ups.

The book's snack and appetizer sections include probiotics-rich snack ideas, easy-to-digest snacks, portable snacks for on-the-go, and dessert recipes that include dairy-free ice cream, fruit-based treats, low-sugar options, gut-soothing gelatin desserts, and baked goods that are acceptable for people with UC. The beverage and smoothie sections include chapters that offer hydrating drinks, anti-inflammatory teas, nutrient-packed smoothies, homemade electrolyte drinks, and guidance on consuming alcohol while using UC.

The book addresses common questions and concerns offers strategies for managing flare-ups and necessary dietary adjustments, addresses food sensitivities and allergies, manages weight loss and malnutrition, and provides advice on traveling and dining out with UC. It also covers long-term dietary management strategies, giving readers the knowledge and skills they need to maintain a healthy diet and effectively manage their condition over time.

CHAPTER ONE

ULCERATIVE COLITIS DIET INTRODUCTION

DEFINITION AND SYNOPSIS

The symptoms of Ulcerative Colitis (UC) include abdominal pain, diarrhea (usually bloody), fatigue, and weight loss. The exact cause of UC is unknown, but it is thought to involve an abnormal immune response triggered by genetic and environmental factors. UC differs from Crohn's disease in that it only affects the innermost lining of the colon, while Crohn's can affect any part of the digestive tract. Ulcerative colitis is a chronic inflammatory bowel disease (IBD) that primarily affects the colon and rectum.

The goal of treatment is to induce and maintain remission, which can vary in duration and intensity from person to person. Knowledge of the nature of UC and its impact on the digestive system is crucial for effectively managing the condition and improving quality of life. UC is managed through a combination of medications to reduce inflammation and control symptoms, as well as lifestyle modifications, including diet modifications. Individuals with UC must work closely with healthcare professionals to monitor their condition and adjust treatment plans as needed.

SIGNS AND PROGNOSIS

Diagnosing ulcerative colitis (UC) usually entails a combination of medical history review, physical examination, blood tests, stool tests to rule out infections, imaging studies such as colonoscopy or sigmoidoscopy, and biopsy of the colon tissue to confirm inflammation. Symptoms of UC can vary widely but commonly include diarrhea (often with blood or pus), abdominal pain and cramping, rectal bleeding, urgency to defecate, fatigue, and unintended weight loss.

Patients exhibiting symptoms suggestive of ulcerative colitis (UC) should seek medical attention as soon as possible to receive an accurate diagnosis and an appropriate treatment plan tailored to their individual needs. Regular monitoring and symptom management are essential aspects of living with UC to minimize complications and improve overall well-being. An early diagnosis is crucial because it allows for the prompt initiation of treatment to control inflammation and manage symptoms effectively. The diagnostic process may require multiple tests and consultations with gastroenterologists or specialists in inflammatory bowel diseases.

REASONS AND DANGER ELEMENTS

While the precise etiology of ulcerative colitis is still unknown, it is thought to be the result of a complex interplay between genetic predisposition, environmental factors, and an aberrant immune response. Genetic studies have revealed specific gene mutations that may heighten the risk of developing ulcerative colitis (UC), especially in those who have a family history of the condition. Environmental factors, including stress, diet, and exposure to specific microbes, may also contribute to the development of UC in susceptible individuals.

Understanding these risk factors can help individuals and healthcare providers identify those at higher risk and implement preventive strategies when possible. Risk factors for developing UC include age (usually diagnosed between the ages of 15 and 30 or after 60), family history of UC or other autoimmune diseases, ethnicity (more common in Caucasians and Ashkenazi Jews), and geographic location (higher incidence in developed countries). Smoking has been identified as a significant risk factor, with smokers being more likely to experience more severe symptoms if they do develop UC.

EFFECTS ON DAY-TO-DAY LIVING

Because of its unpredictable nature and chronic symptoms, ulcerative colitis (UC) can have a significant impact on daily life. UC symptoms such as fatigue, frequent bowel movements, urgency to use the restroom, and abdominal pain can interfere with work, social activities, and overall quality of life. UC can also be emotionally taxing, as living with a chronic illness can exacerbate symptoms of anxiety, depression, and stress. UC management often involves dietary adjustments, scheduling bathroom breaks, and possibly taking medications that have variable side effects.

Despite its challenges, many people with UC can lead fulfilling lives with proper management and support. Strategies like stress management techniques, regular exercise, and maintaining a balanced diet can help minimize symptoms and improve overall well-being. Employers, friends, and family members may need education about the disease to better understand its impact and provide necessary support. Sustaining open communication with healthcare providers and support networks is crucial for coping with the physical and emotional challenges of UC.

DIET IS IMPORTANT FOR MANAGEMENT

Maintaining a food journal can help track symptoms about dietary intake and identify personal triggers. While there is no one-size-fits-all diet for ulcerative colitis, there are dietary principles that can help individuals manage their condition more effectively. These include identifying and avoiding trigger foods that exacerbate symptoms, such as spicy foods, dairy products, caffeine, and high-fiber foods during flare-ups. However, there is no one-size-fits-all diet for UC.

Under the supervision of a healthcare provider or registered dietitian, some individuals with UC may benefit from specific diets such as low-residue diets or exclusion diets. Individuals with UC must collaborate closely with their healthcare team to create a personalized dietary plan that meets their nutritional needs while minimizing symptoms and promoting overall health. A balanced diet rich in nutrients, such as fruits, vegetables, lean proteins, and whole grains, can help maintain gut health and prevent nutritional deficiencies during periods of remission.

Knowing how food affects ulcerative colitis (UC) enables people to make decisions that will improve their quality of life.

CHAPTER TWO

DIETARY INTERVENTIONS FOR ULCERATIVE COLITIS

THE IMPACT OF FOOD ON INFLAMMATION

For people who have ulcerative colitis (UC), diet is very important. Certain foods can cause the gut to become more inflammatory, which can increase symptoms and flare-ups. Foods high in fat, sugar, and processed ingredients can also cause inflammation by upsetting the gut microbiota and inducing an immune response. On the other hand, foods that are considered anti-inflammatory, like fruits, vegetables, lean proteins, and whole grains, can help lower inflammation and improve gut health. Omega-3 fatty acids, which are found in fish and flaxseed, can also help reduce inflammation.

To comprehend the relationship between diet and inflammation, one must be aware of how specific nutrients influence the body's immune response. For instance, foods high in fiber promote regular bowel movements and lessen the burden on the colon; antioxidants found in berries and leafy greens fight oxidative stress; probiotics, which are present in yogurt and fermented foods, can also support gut health by preserving the proper balance of good bacteria; and by concentrating on these dietary components, people with ulcerative colitis can better control their inflammation and enhance their quality of life.

Ultimately, a thoughtful approach to diet can make a significant difference in managing UC symptoms. In addition to food choices, meal timing, and portion control are crucial in managing inflammation. Eating smaller, more frequent meals can prevent overloading the digestive system and reduce inflammation triggers. Staying hydrated with plenty of water and avoiding alcohol and caffeine can also help keep inflammation at bay.

RECOGNIZING FOOD TRIGGERS

To prevent flare-ups and effectively manage symptoms, people with ulcerative colitis must identify common trigger foods, which include dairy products, high-fiber foods, spicy dishes, caffeine, and alcohol. Patients can keep a food diary to track their meals and symptoms, which can help identify specific foods that cause discomfort or exacerbate inflammation. Noting any patterns in flare-ups about food intake allows for more precise dietary adjustments.

Upon identification of trigger foods, it is imperative to either eliminate or minimize their consumption. For example, if dairy products cause problems, it may be beneficial to switch to lactose-free or plant-based alternatives such as almond or soy milk. Similarly, choosing cooked vegetables over raw ones can facilitate easier digestion.

Personalized advice and alternatives can be obtained by consulting with a dietitian, ensuring nutritional needs are met while avoiding problematic foods.

After a period of elimination, another useful tactic is to reintroduce foods one at a time, slowly. This approach, also referred to as an elimination diet, helps determine which foods are safe to eat and which are triggers. During this phase, it's critical to monitor the body's reaction and make necessary adjustments to the diet to balance managing symptoms with having a varied diet.

ADVANTAGES OF A CUSTOMIZED DIET PLAN

For those who suffer from ulcerative colitis, a personalized diet plan has many advantages. Patients can better control their symptoms and lessen the frequency of flare-ups by customizing food choices to meet their needs and triggers. A well-planned diet can supply vital nutrients that support general health and well-being, promoting healing and boosting energy levels. Individual preferences, nutritional needs, and lifestyle factors are taken into consideration, making the plan more sustainable and manageable.

Developing a customized diet plan entails working with medical professionals, such as dietitians and gastroenterologists, who can provide professional advice and assistance. They can assist in developing a balanced meal plan that stays away from triggers and makes sure that enough vitamins, minerals, and other essential nutrients are consumed. This helps manage ulcerative colitis (UC) and prevents nutritional deficiencies that can result from restrictive eating practices.

By offering a stable nutritional foundation, patients may experience fewer side effects from medications and recover from flare-ups more quickly. In general, a personalized diet plan empowers individuals to take control of their condition and improve their quality of life through mindful eating practices. Furthermore, a customized diet plan can increase the efficacy of other treatments for UC, such as medication and lifestyle changes.

UC PATIENTS' NUTRITIONAL REQUIREMENTS

Patients with ulcerative colitis have specific nutritional needs that must be carefully considered to support overall health and manage symptoms. Chronic inflammation and frequent bowel movements can result in deficiencies, so it's important to make sure you're getting enough of key nutrients like protein, vitamins, and minerals. Protein is particularly important for immune function and tissue repair, so lean meats, fish, eggs, and plant-based proteins are valuable additions to the diet. Iron, calcium, and vitamin D are also essential for preventing anemia and supporting bone health.

Supplementation may be required for specific nutrients like vitamin B12 and folate, which can be poorly absorbed in individuals with UC. Including a variety of nutrient-dense foods can help meet these needs while minimizing the risk of flare-ups. For example, choosing cooked vegetables over raw can make them easier to digest and less likely to irritate the gut. Smoothies and pureed soups can be great ways to consume fruits and vegetables without triggering symptoms.

Another crucial component of nutritional care for patients with UC is hydration. Fluid loss and diarrhea can cause dehydration, so, during flare-ups, it's crucial to stay hydrated and think about consuming electrolyte-rich fluids. Reducing inflammation and sugary drinks can also help people stay hydrated.

By emphasizing balanced nutrition and proper hydration, patients with UC can better manage their condition and support their general health.

TYPICAL DIETARY STRATEGIES

Many common dietary approaches are effective in managing symptoms for many individuals with ulcerative colitis (UC). One such approach is the Low FODMAP diet, which involves reducing the intake of fermentable carbohydrates that can cause gas, bloating, and diarrhea; by eliminating specific types of sugars found in certain fruits, vegetables, dairy, and grains, the diet can help identify which foods are safe to consume and which should be avoided. Dietitians can provide guidance when following the Low FODMAP diet.

The Specific Carbohydrate Diet (SCD) is another well-liked strategy that focuses on removing complex carbohydrates that can be challenging to digest and ferment in the gut. The SCD places a strong emphasis on eating simple, natural foods like meat, fish, eggs, vegetables, and some fruits.

It also targets gut healing by reducing the consumption of processed foods and sugars that feed bad bacteria in the gut and reducing inflammation.

Another dietary approach that emphasizes whole, unprocessed foods can help reduce overall inflammation and support better management of UC symptoms is the Anti-Inflammatory Diet, which emphasizes the incorporation of foods known for their anti-inflammatory properties, such as fatty fish, nuts, seeds, olive oil, and plenty of fruits and vegetables. It also encourages the reduction of red meat, processed foods, and refined sugars.

CHAPTER THREE

CRUCIAL ELEMENTS FOR INFLAMMATORY BOWEL DISEASE

FIBER'S SIGNIFICANCE

Insoluble fiber, found in whole grains and vegetables, adds bulk to stool and promotes regularity; soluble fiber, found in foods like oats, apples, and carrots, dissolves in water to form a gel-like substance that can slow digestion and ease symptoms; and for those with ulcerative colitis, starting with low-fiber foods and gradually increasing intake can prevent irritation and flare-ups.

Vegetables can also be cooked or steamed to make them easier to digest and reduce the risk of triggering symptoms.

A diet rich in fiber can also help control the inflammation brought on by ulcerative colitis. Soluble fiber functions as a prebiotics, nourishing the good bacteria in your stomach and reducing inflammation.

Foods high in fiber and omega-3 fatty acids, which have anti-inflammatory qualities, such as flaxseeds and chia seeds, are especially helpful. You can incorporate these seeds into smoothies or baked goods to increase your intake of fiber.

A low-residue diet can help reduce the amount of undigested food passing through the intestines, thereby preventing blockages and alleviating pain. Foods that are low in residue include white rice, bananas, and lean meats; these foods can provide essential nutrients without aggravating symptoms. It is always advisable to speak with a healthcare provider to customize your fiber intake to your unique requirements and tolerance levels.

PROBIOTICS AND PREBIOTICS' ROLES

Probiotics, or live beneficial bacteria, are good for your gut health because they can help restore the balance of the gut microbiome, which is often upset in people with ulcerative colitis. You can find these good bacteria in fermented foods like yogurt, kefir, sauerkraut, and kimchi.

You can also buy probiotics supplements, which are a convenient option for people who find it hard to incorporate fermented foods into their daily diets.

Prebiotics are non-digestible fibers that support the growth of probiotics in the gut. Foods high in prebiotics include garlic, onions, leeks, asparagus, and bananas. Including these foods in your diet can help increase the amount of probiotics in your body and improve your gut health in general. For example, you can add prebiotics to soups and stews or just snack on bananas to get a consistent supply of prebiotics. Synbiotics, or the combination of probiotics and prebiotics, can enhance the benefits of both probiotics and prebiotics.

While probiotics introduce beneficial bacteria, prebiotics make sure these bacteria are well-nourished and able to thrive in the gut environment. Eating a variety of both types of foods regularly can help maintain gut health, reduce symptoms, and improve overall well-being. It's important to monitor your body's response to these foods and make necessary dietary adjustments, consulting a healthcare provider when necessary.

MINERALS AND VITAMINS TO PAY ATTENTION TO

Because ulcerative colitis can cause inflammation and frequent diarrhea, patients need to ensure they are getting enough of certain vitamins and minerals. For example, vitamin D, which is found in foods like fatty fish, fortified dairy products, and supplements, as well as sunshine exposure, is essential for immune system function and bone health. Low vitamin D levels are common in ulcerative colitis patients, so it is important to monitor and supplement as needed.

Iron is another important mineral that needs to be taken care of. Iron deficiency anemia can be caused by chronic blood loss from intestinal bleeding. Foods high in iron, like lean meats, spinach, and fortified cereals, can help maintain healthy iron levels; however, those with significant deficiencies may need to take iron supplements.

Iron absorption can be improved by pairing iron-rich foods with sources of vitamin C, such as citrus fruits or bell peppers.

Since ulcerative colitis can affect the absorption of these vitamins, including sources like eggs, dairy products, leafy greens, and fortified cereals in your diet is beneficial. B12 supplements might be required, especially if you follow a vegetarian or vegan diet. Regular blood tests can help monitor levels and ensure you are meeting your nutritional needs. B vitamins, particularly B12, and folate, are crucial for energy production and maintaining nerve health.

HYDRATION: ITS ADVANTAGES

Although frequent diarrhea can cause dehydration, drinking plenty of fluids throughout the day supports overall bodily functions and helps maintain electrolyte balance; water is the best choice, but electrolyte-rich beverages like sports drinks or coconut water can also be helpful, especially during flare-ups; herbal teas and broths can provide additional nutrients and hydration without irritating the digestive tract.

Hydrating foods like cucumbers, watermelon, and oranges can contribute to your overall fluid intake. These foods not only provide water but also essential vitamins and minerals that support overall health.

A simple way to check your level of hydration is to look at the color of your urine; light yellow urine usually indicates adequate hydration. Dehydration can exacerbate symptoms and lead to complications like kidney stones or urinary tract infections.

Apart from drinking plenty of water and eating foods high in hydration, it's critical to control your electrolyte levels. Diarrhea causes the loss of electrolytes such as sodium, potassium, and magnesium, which can be restored through food or supplements to help sustain muscle function and avoid cramps. Foods high in these electrolytes include bananas, avocados, and leafy greens.

Before making any major dietary or hydration-related changes, always speak with your healthcare provider to make sure your plan is appropriate for you.

SUPPLEMENTS FOR EXTRA ASSISTANCE

Probiotic supplements containing strains like Lactobacillus and Bifidobacterium can help restore gut flora balance and reduce symptoms. Omega-3 fatty acids, found in fish oil supplements, have anti-inflammatory properties that can help reduce inflammation in the digestive tract. These supplements can be a beneficial addition to a diet already rich in omega-3s from sources like salmon and flaxseeds. Supplements can play a supportive role in managing ulcerative colitis by addressing specific nutritional deficiencies and promoting gut health.

A sufficient intake of these nutrients is essential for long-term health. Vitamin D deficiency is common in people with ulcerative colitis, and it plays a role in immune function and bone health. The appropriate dosage for an individual with ulcerative colitis should be determined based on the results of blood tests and under the supervision of a healthcare provider. Similarly, calcium supplements may be required, particularly for those taking corticosteroids, which can affect bone density.

The potential anti-inflammatory effects of herbal supplements, like aloe vera and turmeric, have been studied. Turmeric's curcumin, which has been shown to reduce inflammation, can help soothe the digestive tract, but aloe vera juice should be used with caution as it may have laxative effects. It's important to talk to your healthcare provider before beginning any new supplement regimen to make sure it is safe, appropriate for your particular condition, and won't interfere with any medications you may be taking.

CHAPTER FOUR

CREATING A DIET PLAN FOR ULCERATIVE COLITIS

CREATING DIETARY OBJECTIVES

The first step in managing ulcerative colitis (UC) is establishing dietary goals. To start, speak with a registered dietitian or your healthcare provider to find out what your individual nutritional needs are. They can also help you understand the significance of avoiding trigger foods while making sure you get the nutrients you need.

Your goals should include maintaining a healthy weight, making sure you get enough vitamins and minerals, and managing symptoms with a balanced diet. Make sure to include anti-inflammatory foods like lean proteins, omega-3 fatty acids, and lots of fruits and vegetables in your diet, while avoiding high-fiber foods during flare-ups.

Starting a food diary is a good way to identify foods that trigger you or make you feel a certain way after eating.

You can use this information to identify trigger foods and to better understand how your body responds to different foods. Based on your food diary data, you can create SMART goals, such as aiming to eat at least two servings of low-fiber vegetables per day or substituting fruit for sugary snacks three times a week. You can also modify your goals based on ongoing observations and any changes in your symptoms or overall health.

Celebrate small victories and remain patient, as managing UC through diet is an ongoing process that requires consistency and dedication.

Regular check-ins with your dietitian or healthcare provider can help you stay on track and make necessary adjustments. Regularly review and adjust your dietary goals to ensure they remain relevant to your condition and overall health. UC symptoms and triggers can change over time, so it's essential to stay flexible and responsive to your body's needs.

MAKING A WELL-COMPOSED MEAL PLAN

A well-rounded meal plan for ulcerative colitis consists of foods that promote general health and reduce symptoms. To begin, portion your plate into lean protein, healthy fat, and easily digested carbohydrate servings.

Lean protein options include chicken, fish, eggs, and tofu; for healthy fats, choose avocado, olive oil, and flaxseeds; for carbohydrates, choose low-fiber options like white rice, peeled potatoes, and refined grains during flare-ups, and gradually reintroduce whole grains during remission.

Aim to include probiotics-rich foods, like yogurt and kefir, to support gut health. Plan your meals around nutrient-dense foods to ensure you get all the vitamins and minerals you need. Include a variety of fruits and vegetables, but be aware of those that may cause discomfort. Cooking techniques like steaming, boiling, or roasting can make vegetables easier to digest.

Hydration is also important; drink lots of water throughout the day and stay away from sugary drinks and caffeine, which can irritate the digestive tract.

Plan your meals and store them in portion-sized containers for convenience. This will save time and ensure that you always have UC-friendly meals on hand, reducing the risk of reaching for unhealthy options during busy days. Create a weekly menu that includes breakfast, lunch, dinner, and snacks. This will help ensure you have a variety of meals and reduce the temptation to eat foods that may trigger symptoms.

TIPS FOR GROCERY SHOPPING

A UC-friendly diet requires effective grocery shopping. Begin by making a comprehensive shopping list based on your meal plan. Add a range of lean proteins, easily digested carbohydrates, healthy fats, and fresh produce. Give anti-inflammatory foods a top priority and stay away from items that are known to trigger symptoms. Shop the perimeter of the store, where fresh, whole foods are usually found, to avoid impulse purchases.

Choose a variety of low-fiber fruits and vegetables (bananas, melons, avocados, cooked or peeled carrots) when shopping for produce. Lean meat, poultry, and fish are good sources of protein. If you purchase packaged foods, choose items with few ingredients and steer clear of additives that can exacerbate UC symptoms. Whole foods are usually the best choice, but if you must have convenience items, look for those that are labeled as organic, non-GMO, and preservative-free.

Make your grocery shopping more efficient by going to farmers' markets or health food stores; these places usually have fresher, higher-quality products.

Buying in bulk can also help you save money and guarantee that you always have UC-friendly staples on hand. Stock your pantry with staples like pasta, white rice, canned tuna, and low-fiber snacks. Making a list and following it will help you manage your UC more effectively and encourage healthier eating habits in general.

EXAMINING NUTRITION LABELS

One of the most important skills in managing ulcerative colitis is reading food labels because it helps you steer clear of ingredients that could set off flare-ups. Look for ingredients like high-fiber grains, lactose, gluten, and artificial additives on the ingredient list. Products with long lists of unpronounceable ingredients are processed and may contain harmful chemicals; instead, look for products with short, recognizable ingredient lists that emphasize whole foods.

The nutritional information on the label should be closely examined. You should look for information on the amount of dietary fiber, sugars, and unhealthy fats, as these can affect your symptoms.

If you experience flare-ups, choose low-fiber foods and then gradually reintroduce higher-fiber foods once your condition stabilizes. You should also look for products with lower sodium content, and whenever possible, choose fresh or minimally processed foods.

Food labels can contain misleading information about serving sizes; for example, the nutritional values listed are frequently for a single serving, which may be smaller than the portion you typically consume. This can result in unintentional overconsumption of irritants; to prevent this, measure your portions based on the information provided on serving sizes and modify your intake accordingly. By effectively understanding and utilizing food labels, you can make educated dietary decisions that will help you better manage your UC symptoms.

ORGANIZING MEALS FOR CONVENIENCE

Meal prep is a useful tactic for ulcerative colitis management because it guarantees that you always have wholesome, symptom-friendly meals available. To begin, schedule a specific time each week to plan and cook your meals. Select recipes that support your dietary objectives and are simple to digest. By cooking in bulk, you can cut down on time and anxiety during hectic workdays.

Prepare basic ingredients like cooked chicken, steamed vegetables, and grains that can be combined to create different meals.

Investing in freezer- and microwave-safe storage containers is a great idea. Portion meals into these containers so that you always have balanced servings on hand. Label each container with the contents and the date so you can keep an eye on its freshness. Freezing some meals is a great way to have options available for weeks when you might not have time to cook; soups, stews, and casseroles work particularly well.

Plan your meal prep by meal type: breakfasts, lunches, dinners, and snacks. For breakfast, think about things like scrambled eggs with avocado or overnight oats with UC-friendly toppings. For lunch and dinner, think about things like grilled chicken with rice and steamed veggies. For snacks, think about portioned servings of fruit, yogurt, or cheese. Eating a variety of meals prepared ahead of time keeps you on track with your diet and lessens the chance that you'll eat trigger foods.

CHAPTER FIVE

GETTING STARTED

FUNDAMENTAL COOKING METHODS

Learning these foundational cooking techniques will lay the groundwork for more complex cooking later on. When starting to cook for an ulcerative colitis diet, it's important to start with basic methods like boiling, steaming, and baking, which preserve nutrients and are easy on the digestive system. For example, boiling vegetables can soften fibers and make them easier to digest, while steaming retains most of the vitamins and minerals. Baking meats and fish allows you to avoid added fats and create meals that are satisfying and healthful.

Sautéing with healthy fats—using olive oil or coconut oil—adds flavor and healthy nutrients without upsetting the stomach. Sautéing should be done at a moderate heat to prevent burning the oil and releasing toxic compounds.

Sautéing vegetables—like bell peppers, zucchini, and carrots—lightly improve their flavor and digestibility. Adding fresh herbs and spices to your food also adds variety and health benefits.

A high-quality blender is a worthwhile investment, enabling you to create a variety of UC-friendly meals. For instance, blending cooked vegetables with a bit of broth can create a soothing, nutrient-rich soup. Similarly, pureeing fruits for smoothies ensures you get the vitamins and minerals you need without excessively taxing your digestive system. Blending and pureeing foods can also be beneficial for individuals with UC. Smoothies, soups, and purees are easier on the digestive system and can be loaded with nutrients.

ESSENTIAL KITCHEN ITEMS FOR UC-FRIENDLY COOKING

Having the proper tools in your kitchen is essential for successful UC-friendly cooking. Non-stick cookware reduces the need for excessive oils and fats. A good set of knives is necessary for safely and efficiently chopping ingredients; they also help retain the integrity of the food, making it easier to digest and more palatable.

Purchasing a high-quality food processor or blender can also simplify meal preparation. These appliances are ideal for producing creamy, easily digested soups, smoothies, and purees.

They let you blend multiple ingredients into a single, nutrient-dense meal that may be less taxing on the digestive system. Moreover, owning an instant pot or slow cooker can be immensely helpful for producing flavorful, soft meals quickly, which is ideal for hectic days or times when you need to prepare meals ahead of time.

Another must-have for a UC-friendly kitchen is storage containers. Choose airtight, BPA-free containers to keep your ingredients fresh and avoid contamination; glass containers work best because they don't absorb chemicals into your food and can be used for both reheating and storage; a well-stocked pantry with clearly labeled containers can also help you find what you need quickly, which will make cooking easier and less stressful.

SAFE FOOD HANDLING PROCEDURES

To ensure that your food is safe to eat, it is important to follow safe food handling procedures. To start, wash your hands well with soap and water before handling any food. This small but effective step can cut down on the likelihood that harmful bacteria will find their way into your food. You should also make sure that all surfaces and utensils are clean before using them, and sanitize cutting boards—especially after chopping raw meat or fish—to prevent cross-contamination.

To prevent cross-contamination when handling raw ingredients, keep meats and vegetables apart; use different cutting boards and knives for raw meat and produce; store raw meat at the bottom of the refrigerator to prevent juices from dripping onto other foods; and store cooked and raw foods at the proper temperatures to prevent the growth of harmful bacteria.

For example, keep your freezer at 0°F (-18°C) and your refrigerator at or below 40°F (4°C).

Another crucial procedure is cooking food to the proper temperature. To guarantee that meats are cooked through and reach safe internal temperatures to destroy any harmful bacteria, use a food thermometer. For instance, poultry should be cooked to an internal temperature of 165°F (74°C), and ground meats should be cooked to 160°F (71°C). You should also reheat leftovers to at least 165°F (74°C) to ensure that any potential bacteria are destroyed and your food is safe to eat.

ADVICE ON HOW TO LOWER FOOD CONTAMINATION
Buying fresh, high-quality produce is the first step towards reducing food contamination. Fruits and vegetables that are bruised or otherwise blemished are more vulnerable to bacterial growth. When shopping for meat, choose cuts that are well-sealed and do not smell bad—these are signs of freshness. If at all possible, purchase organic to avoid pesticides and other chemicals that can be hard on the digestive system.

Another crucial step is to store your ingredients properly. Keep your pantry cool and dry, check expiration dates frequently, and arrange your pantry so that older items are used first to minimize the risk of consuming expired foods. Perishable items, such as meat, dairy, and produce, should always be kept in the refrigerator.

Keeping your kitchen clean is essential. You should routinely clean countertops, sinks, and other frequently touched surfaces. You should also wash and sanitize all utensils, cutting boards, and appliances after cooking. Finally, you should refrigerate leftovers as soon as possible to reduce the risk of bacterial contamination and make sure your food is safe to eat.

MODIFYING RECIPES TO MAKE MEALS UC-FRIENDLY

If you want to modify a recipe to make it more UC-friendly, you should swap out high-fiber vegetables for lower-fiber ones like peeled carrots, zucchini, and squash. You can also switch out dairy, which can be hard for some UC sufferers to digest, for lactose-free or plant-based alternatives like almond or coconut milk. These small changes can have a big impact on how well your body handles the meal.

Lean protein intake is another key adjustment. Select fish and lean meats, such as turkey or chicken breast, that are high in omega-3 fatty acids, and have anti-inflammatory qualities. Steer clear of processed meats and bake, grill, or steam instead of fry to cut down on added fat. Use tofu and eggs as substitute protein sources, which can be more easily digested while still offering the required amount of protein.

Ultimately, tweaking cooking techniques can help make recipes more UC-friendly. For example, slow-cooking soups and stews breaks down ingredients into more easily digested forms; pureeing vegetables into soups and sauces can help create smoother, less-aggressive textures; and experimenting with herbs and spices rather than depending solely on heavy seasonings and sauces can add flavor without upsetting your digestive tract.

CHAPTER SIX

MEAL PLANNING AND PREPARATION

COMPREHENDING MACRONUTRIENTS

Proteins play a vital role in tissue repair and immune function, which is especially important for people with ulcerative colitis (UC), as they frequently experience inflammation and potential damage to the intestinal lining. Lean meats, fish, eggs, and plant-based options like beans and tofu are good sources of protein because they are gentler on the digestive system. Macronutrients, which include proteins, carbohydrates, and fats, are necessary for the body's overall function and health.

The body uses carbs as its main energy source, so for people with UC, it's important to choose easily digested carbohydrates to prevent symptoms from occurring. Choose refined pasta, white rice, and potatoes instead of whole grains because they are less likely to irritate the digestive tract.

Keeping a balance between simple and complex carbohydrates helps keep energy levels stable without putting too much strain on the intestines.

Healthy fats, like those in avocados, olive oil, and fatty fish like salmon, should be prioritized because they help reduce inflammation, which can be especially helpful for UC patients. Trans fats and high-fat processed foods can exacerbate symptoms and cause flare-ups. Fats are essential for the absorption of vitamins and long-term energy.

PROTEIN, CARBOHYDRATE, AND FAT EQUILIBRIUM

A balanced meal plan for UC requires a careful distribution of macronutrients throughout the day. A good breakfast consists of a combination of carbohydrates and protein, like scrambled eggs with a side of white toast, which helps to kickstart metabolism and sustains energy. Mid-morning snacks, such as a small yogurt or banana, help to stabilize blood sugar levels.

Lunch should consist of lean proteins and moderate carbohydrates, such as grilled chicken with mashed potatoes and steamed carrots; this combination makes sure the body gets the nutrients it needs without stressing the digestive tract. You should also include a small amount of healthy fats, like olive oil drizzled over vegetables, to help absorb the nutrients and reduce inflammation.

A variety of vegetables helps ensure fiber intake without being harsh on the digestive tract; adjusting the balance of macronutrients based on daily activities and energy needs ensures that the body is adequately nourished without triggering UC symptoms. Dinner can be lighter, emphasizing easily digested proteins and carbohydrates, such as baked fish with rice and sautéed zucchini.

FIBER'S SIGNIFICANCE AND HOW TO INCLUDE IT

For UC patients, soluble fiber—found in foods like oats, apples, and carrots—can help regulate bowel movements and reduce symptoms. It also forms a gel-like substance in the gut that slows digestion and can prevent diarrhea, a common symptom of UC. Fiber is essential for digestive health, but UC patients must choose the right kind and amount of fiber.

Fiber must be added to the diet gradually to prevent overtaxing the digestive system. Smoothies made from blended fruits and vegetables are another gentle way to increase fiber intake without irritating the digestive tract. Start with small portions of cooked vegetables, like peeled zucchini or carrots, and gradually increase the amount.

Eat more well-cooked, peeled, and seedless fruits and vegetables; high-fiber foods that can be harsh on the intestines, like raw vegetables, nuts, seeds, and whole grains, should be avoided, especially during flare-ups. Even small amounts of fiber at each meal can help maintain digestive health and help manage UC symptoms more effectively.

EXAMPLE MEAL SCHEDULES FOR VARIOUS UC STAGES

A typical day might start with scrambled eggs and white toast for breakfast, followed by a grilled chicken salad with cooked vegetables for lunch, and baked fish with rice and steamed carrots for dinner.

Snacks could include yogurt, bananas, and applesauce. Meal plans for UC patients should be customized to different stages of the disease, whether in remission or during a flare-up.

A simple, water-based oatmeal for breakfast, a ripe banana for a midmorning snack, boiled chicken and mashed potatoes for lunch, and plain rice and baked, peeled apples for dinner are all good ways to minimize symptoms during a flare-up. Raw vegetables, high-fiber foods, and anything too spicy or fatty should also be avoided.

Starting with cooked, peeled vegetables and working your way up to lean proteins and mild carbohydrates, transitioning between stages entails gradually reintroducing more variety as symptoms subside. Keeping a food diary can help identify any foods that trigger symptoms, allowing for a more individualized approach to meal planning.

CHANGING MEAL PLANS IN RESPONSE TO SYMPTOMS

UC must be effectively managed by modifying meal plans in response to symptoms. If diarrhea is present, concentrate on low-fiber, easily-digested foods like white rice, plain pasta, and applesauce.

These foods help solidify stools and lessen bowel movements. Drink plenty of fluids to stay hydrated because diarrhea can cause dehydration.

Increase your intake of soluble fiber by eating more oatmeal, peeled apples, and carrots. You can also help ease constipation by focusing on gentle sources of fiber, avoiding high-fiber foods that can cause bloating or discomfort, and staying hydrated. You can also include healthy fats like avocado or olive oil in your diet.

Small, frequent meals are often easier to tolerate than large ones; during periods of severe symptoms, such as cramping or pain, choose bland, non-irritating foods like boiled chicken, mashed potatoes, and plain rice; close observation of symptoms and diet adjustments help manage UC more effectively, relieving symptoms and accelerating healing.

RECIPES FOR BREAKFAST

SMOOTHIES TO PROMOTE DIGESTIVE HEALTH

Smoothies are a great way to start the day and support gut health, especially for people who are managing ulcerative colitis. Start with a base that is easy on the stomach, like almond milk or coconut water, and then add nutrient-dense fruits like bananas, blueberries, and papayas, which are full of vitamins and antioxidants. If you want to add even more nutrition, you can add a handful of leafy greens, like spinach or kale, which are high in fiber and essential nutrients but blend smoothly without tasting strongly.

Blend all the ingredients until smooth, making sure there are no chunks that could be hard to digest. Add gut-friendly ingredients like ginger (which has anti-inflammatory properties) and a tablespoon of chia or flaxseeds for added fiber and omega-3 fatty acids. If you want to up the probiotics content of your smoothie, you can also add a spoonful of dairy-free yogurt or a splash of kefir.

Try experimenting with different combinations to find what works best for you, and always start with small portions to ensure your digestive system can handle the ingredients. Supplements like glutamine powder, which supports gut lining health, or a probiotics powder to increase beneficial bacteria in your gut can make your smoothie even more beneficial for gut health.

SIMPLE-TO-DIGEST OATMEAL RECIPES

For those who suffer from ulcerative colitis, oatmeal is a calming and adaptable breakfast choice. To prevent any possible sensitivity, start with gluten-free oats and cook them in water or almond milk until they become creamy. You can add mashed bananas or applesauce for natural sweetness and to aid in digestion. These fruits also contain vital vitamins and minerals that are easy on the stomach.

A spoonful of pumpkin puree or a handful of finely grated carrots can be added for extra flavor and nutrients; these are both high in fiber and vitamins but soft enough to digest easily; a dash of vanilla extract or a sprinkle of cinnamon can add flavor without adding any harsh ingredients; instead of adding nuts or seeds directly to the oatmeal—which can be hard to digest—try adding a spoonful of nut butter, which mixes well into the oatmeal and provides healthy fats.

Always serve your oatmeal warm, as hot food is generally easier to digest than cold. Experiment with different flavors and textures to keep your breakfast interesting while ensuring it remains easy on your digestive system. Or, add a scoop of sensitive-tummy-friendly protein powder or mix in a beaten egg while cooking to create a custard-like texture.

HIGH-PROTEIN EGG RECIPES

Eggs are an excellent source of protein and can be cooked in ways that are easy on the digestive system. To start your day, make a simple dish of scrambled eggs in a non-stick pan with a tiny bit of olive or coconut oil. Whisk the eggs well and cook on low heat to prevent browning, which can make the eggs more difficult to digest.

You can also add some finely chopped spinach or zucchini for extra nutrients without packing on the pounds.

To keep the egg whites and yolks soft and easier to digest, another simple option is a soft-boiled or poached egg, which can be served over a slice of gluten-free toast or alongside steamed vegetables. To add some variation, beat eggs with finely chopped vegetables, such as bell peppers and mushrooms, pour the mixture into a muffin tin, and bake until set. These can be prepared ahead of time and reheated for a healthy and quick breakfast.

A simple and well-cooked egg dish will ensure that it provides a nutritious and easily digestible start to your day. If you like omelets, try making one with a combination of egg whites and a few whole eggs for a lighter option. Stuff your omelet with UC-friendly vegetables and a small amount of dairy-free cheese for extra flavor. Avoid adding heavy meats or too many spices as these can be hard on your digestive system.

WAFFLES & PANCAKES THAT ARE UC-FRIENDLY

Pancakes and waffles can still be enjoyed by those who have ulcerative colitis, but they will require some adjustments. To start, use gluten-free flour blends, as these are easier on the stomach. Mix the flour with almond or coconut milk, beaten egg, and a small amount of baking powder to make a light and fluffy batter. Don't use too much sugar; instead, use natural sweeteners like mashed bananas or unsweetened applesauce.

For pancakes, use the same batter but cook in a waffle iron until crisp but tender; serve with a drizzle of pure maple syrup or a topping of fresh berries, avoiding heavy or overly processed toppings. Cook on a non-stick griddle with a small amount of coconut oil to ensure even cooking and prevent sticking. Pancakes should be small and thin to make digestion easier.

Always make sure your pancakes and waffles are thoroughly cooked to prevent any potential digestive issues.

Enjoy these treats in moderation and always keep an eye on how your body reacts to new ingredients. To increase the nutritional value, consider adding a spoonful of ground flaxseeds or chia seeds to the batter. These seeds are high in omega-3 fatty acids and fiber but blend well without affecting the texture.

OPTIONS FOR DAIRY-FREE YOGURT

For people with ulcerative colitis, dairy-free yogurt is a great breakfast choice because it has a creamy texture without the possible irritants associated with dairy. Opt for yogurts made from almond milk, coconut milk, or soy milk, as these are generally less harsh on the digestive system. Look for varieties that have probiotics or live cultures, as these can help support gut health. Steer clear of yogurts that have added sugars or artificial sweeteners, as these can aggravate symptoms.

Add some gentle, nutrient-dense toppings to your yogurt, such as sliced bananas, blueberries, or a spoonful of pureed fruit; these fruits are high in vitamins and antioxidants and easy to digest.

If you want to add even more texture and nutrition, you can also mix in a small amount of gluten-free granola or finely chopped nuts (just make sure the nuts are small and easy to chew) or a spoonful of chia or flaxseeds, which blend well into the yogurt and offer extra fiber and omega-3 fatty acids.

A visually appealing and satisfying breakfast that is easy on the stomach can be made by layering dairy-free yogurt with soft fruits and a drizzle of honey or maple syrup for natural sweetness. Try different flavor combinations and see what works best for you; always start with small portions to ensure your digestive system can handle the ingredients comfortably.

RECIPES FOR LUNCH

SIMPLE AND LIGHT SALADS

An ulcerative colitis diet must include light and simple salads that provide nutrients without inflaming the body. Begin with a base of vitamin-rich, easily digestible leafy greens, like spinach or kale; add vibrant vegetables, like carrots, bell peppers, and cucumbers, for extra fiber and antioxidants; add lean proteins, like grilled chicken or tofu, for flavor and nutrition; and add healthy fats, like avocado or a drizzle of olive oil, to improve satiety and facilitate the absorption of nutrients.

Along with supporting gut health, these salads are a refreshing and nourishing option for any mealtime, ensuring you stay on track with your dietary needs while enjoying delicious and nutritious meals. For a satisfying crunch, sprinkle with seeds or nuts (if tolerated), such as pumpkin seeds or almonds. Keep dressings simple and homemade using ingredients like olive oil, lemon juice, and herbs to avoid additives and preservatives that may irritate the gut. Remember to wash vegetables thoroughly and consider prepping salads in advance for convenience during flare-ups.

HEALTHY BROTHS & SOUPS

Comforting and easily digestible options for people with ulcerative colitis are nourishing soups and broths. Prepare a base of homemade bone broth or vegetable broth, simmered to extract maximum nutrients without additives or excess sodium. Add mild vegetables, like potatoes, carrots, and zucchini, cooked until tender to aid in digestion.

Add lean proteins, like turkey or shredded chicken that provide essential amino acids without exacerbating symptoms.

Add anti-inflammatory herbs and spices like parsley, ginger, and turmeric to boost flavor and nutritional value. Steer clear of heavy creams and seasonings that can exacerbate flare-ups. Soups can be batch-cooked and frozen in portion sizes for easy and quick meals during the week or for flare-ups. These soups and broths are comforting and nourishing, perfect for a light lunch or a calming dinner.

SANDWICHES AND WRAPS WITH LEAN PROTEIN

For an easy and portable ulcerative colitis-friendly meal option, try lean protein wraps and sandwiches. Start with a soft, easily digested wrap or bread (preferably whole grain or gluten-free if necessary).

Select lean proteins like turkey, grilled chicken, or tofu, which provide essential nutrients without being overly fattening or containing additives. Add fresh veggies, such as lettuce, tomatoes, and cucumbers, for fiber and vitamins, to improve texture and nutritional value.

Whether packed for lunch or enjoyed at home, these wraps and sandwiches can be customized to personal taste preferences and dietary needs, making them versatile for any meal of the day. For added flavor and healthy fats that support satiety and nutrient absorption, consider spreads like hummus or avocado.

Steer clear of high-fat or spicy condiments that may trigger symptoms.

EASY GRAIN BOWLS

A base of cooked grains, like quinoa, brown rice, or millet, which provide fiber and essential nutrients without aggravating symptoms, makes for a nutrient-dense meal that can be customized to fit an ulcerative colitis diet. Cooked vegetables, like steamed broccoli, roasted sweet potatoes, or sautéed spinach, add vitamins and minerals that support digestive health.

Add lean proteins (grilled fish, chickpeas, or lean beef) to provide the amino acids needed for overall health and muscle repair. Drizzle a bit of olive oil or sliced avocado on top to add flavor and increase fullness. You can also add herbs and spices (turmeric, basil, or cilantro) for extra taste and anti-inflammatory properties. These grain bowls are incredibly simple to make ahead of time and keep in the refrigerator for weeknight meals that are satisfying and well-balanced.

SIDE DISHES MADE WITH VEGETABLES

An ulcerative colitis diet must include a variety of colorful vegetables, such as steamed broccoli, roasted Brussels sprouts, or sautéed green beans, which offer essential nutrients and antioxidants. Cook vegetables until they are tender to aid in digestion and enhance nutrient absorption. Vegetable-based side dishes are an essential part of an ulcerative colitis diet, providing fiber, vitamins, and minerals without triggering inflammation.

Use herbs and spices like thyme, garlic powder, or rosemary to add flavor without upsetting the stomach. Steer clear of heavy sauces or overly seasoning, as these can exacerbate symptoms. These side dishes are great as snacks or as a side dish to main courses; they are a tasty and nutrient-dense addition to any diet that is ulcerative colitis-friendly. By utilizing seasonal and fresh produce, you can make tasty side dishes that promote overall health and digestive health.

RECIPES FOR DINNER

PASTA DISHES THAT ARE UC-FRIENDLY

To make pasta dishes that are UC-friendly, select ingredients that are easy on the digestive system and still offer satisfying flavors and textures. For example, choose gluten-free pasta varieties made from rice or quinoa, which are easier to digest. Serve these with light sauces made from olive oil, fresh herbs, and low-acid tomatoes. Steer clear of heavy cream-based sauces or sauces that are highly spiced, as these can aggravate symptoms. Add lean proteins, such as grilled chicken or tofu, for extra nutrition without added fat. Make sure to cook pasta according to exact times to preserve pasta integrity, as overcooked pasta can be more difficult to digest.

RICH STEWS AND CASSEROLES

For an ulcerative colitis diet, rich stews and casseroles should be made using slow-cooking methods that break down tough fibers and facilitate digestion.

Lean meat or poultry cuts should be cooked until they are tender, enhancing flavors with herbs and mild spices instead of heavy sauces. Low-residue vegetables, like carrots, potatoes (sans skin), and bell peppers, provide extra nutrients without being overly fibrous. Grains, like quinoa or white rice, can be added for a hearty, nourishing texture that is easy on the stomach. Low-residue vegetables, like carrots, potatoes (sans skin), and bell peppers should be used for added nutrients without being too high in fiber.

OPTIONS FOR GRILLED AND BAKED FISH

Because grilled fish is high in protein and contains omega-3 fatty acids, which can help reduce inflammation, it's a great option for ulcerative colitis-friendly dinners. Mildly flavored fish, like tilapia, cod, or salmon, is easier to digest. Marinate fish in simple, acid-free mixtures like olive oil, lemon juice, and herbs before grilling or baking to enhance flavors without irritating the digestive tract. Serve fish with steamed vegetables or a side dish of mashed sweet potatoes for added nutrition and ease of digestion. Steer clear of heavy sauces or fried preparations, as they can aggravate symptoms. Cook fish thoroughly and gently to ensure it stays tender and digestible.

VEGETARIAN DINNER IDEAS

When coming up with vegetarian dinner ideas for ulcerative colitis, it's important to prioritize plant-based proteins and easily digestible vegetables. Legumes, tofu, and chickpeas are good examples of protein sources that are high in nutrients and fiber without being too harsh on the stomach.

You should also use herbs, garlic, and ginger to season dishes simply; cooked vegetables, such as spinach, squash, or eggplant, are softer and less fibrous. You should also make vegetable-based soups or stir-fries that you can adjust with mild herbs and spices to your taste preferences. Finally, try serving different grains as side dishes to add some diversity and texture.

COMFORT FOOD FOR FLARE-UPS

Well-cooked, mashed potatoes or sweet potatoes seasoned with olive oil and herbs make a comforting side dish. Make chicken or turkey broth-based soups with soft vegetables like carrots and celery to aid in digestion. Include soft, bland grains like oatmeal or white rice to help soothe the stomach. Steer clear of high-fat, spicy, or fried foods to prevent discomfort. Use gentle cooking techniques like steaming, baking, or boiling to preserve food integrity and facilitate digestion. Eating small, frequent meals can also help manage symptoms during flare-ups while ensuring adequate nutrition is received.

These strategies emphasize wholesome, easily digestible ingredients and cooking techniques to promote digestive health and general well-being, to make meal preparation easier for persons who are managing ulcerative colitis.

RECIPES FOR SNACKS AND APPETIZERS

SNACKS GOOD FOR THE STOMACH

Finding gut-friendly snacks is essential for ulcerative colitis (UC). These snacks are easy on the stomach, supporting both nutrition and comfort. Try low-fiber fruits, like bananas or melons, which are easier to digest. Greek yogurt is another great option, known for its probiotics properties and calming effects. If you want to add some protein and healthy fats, top some rice cakes with almond butter for a satisfying crunch without making your stomach feel full.

While hummus with gluten-free crackers offers a combination of protein and fiber, supporting digestive health without causing discomfort, try boiling potatoes with a sprinkle of olive oil and herbs for those who are craving savory options. Start with small portions to gauge tolerance levels and adjust ingredients based on personal preferences. These snacks not only nourish but also support a balanced diet conducive to managing UC symptoms effectively.

SIMPLE-TO-PROCESS APPETIZERS

Making appetizers that are easy on the stomach is crucial for those who suffer from ulcerative colitis. Clear soups and broths are a good place to start because they are warming and hydrating and are also simple to digest. A vegetable broth made with soft-cooked vegetables, such as carrots and zucchini, can be calming and full of nutrients. If you're looking for something lighter, mashed avocado on rice crackers has a creamy texture and healthy fats.

A satisfying appetizer that is low in fiber and high in protein is sliced bite-sized pieces of poached or grilled chicken breast, served with steamed vegetables or a small serving of quinoa for a balanced meal. Steer clear of heavy sauces or spices that could cause discomfort. Rice paper rolls stuffed with shredded chicken, lettuce, and cucumber make a light and satisfying appetizer that not only promotes digestive ease but also guarantees a flavorful start to any meal without sacrificing nutritional value.

IDEAS FOR PROBIOTIC-RICH SNACKS

The addition of probiotics-rich snacks to the diet can help individuals with ulcerative colitis by lowering inflammation and promoting gut health. One such snack is yogurt parfaits topped with fresh berries and chia seeds, which not only improves digestive health but also provides vital antioxidants and omega-3 fatty acids. Another great snack is kefir, a fermented dairy product that tastes good and is full of probiotics that help maintain a healthy gut microbiome.

Try homemade kimchi or sauerkraut, which are traditional fermented foods high in probiotics. Serve them with rice cakes or gluten-free crackers for a filling snack.

Smoothies made with yogurt or kefir, spinach, and pineapple are a cool way to get probiotics into your diet while maintaining optimal nutrient intake. Try blending different flavors to find ones that you enjoy while also supporting digestive wellness.

FAST AND WHOLESOME DIPS

For those with ulcerative colitis, making quick and nutritious dips means convenience without sacrificing nutrition. Start with guacamole, which is made with mashed avocado, lime juice, and a little salt. Rich in fiber and healthy fats, this dip eases digestion and promotes satiety. It goes well with carrot sticks or cucumber slices as a light snack. Greek yogurt-based dips with herbs and garlic add a creamy texture and probiotics benefits that are perfect for improving gut health.

Dips such as hummus, which is made from chickpeas blended with tahini, lemon juice, and olive oil, are high in protein and can help with digestive comfort. They taste great with gluten-free pita bread or celery sticks for a satisfying crunch. Almond butter, when combined with a little honey and cinnamon, is a dairy-free alternative that is sweet and nutrient-dense, high in healthy fats, and rich in protein.

ON-THE-GO PORTABLE SNACKS

To manage ulcerative colitis and lead an active lifestyle, it's important to find portable snacks that are easy on the digestive system. Try making homemade granola bars from oats, nuts, and dried fruits; these bars give you sustained energy without overwhelming your digestive tract. Trail mix is a convenient snack option that is high in protein and healthy fats; choose unsweetened dried fruits to avoid excess sugar.

A portable snack that is simple to make and carry is rice cakes spread with nut butter or topped with avocado slices. These snacks offer a combination of carbohydrates, protein, and healthy fats that support energy levels throughout the day. Hard-boiled eggs that are seasoned with a little salt and pepper are another portable option that is high in protein and essential nutrients. You can pack these with sliced fruit or vegetables for a balanced snack on the go.

DESSERT RECIPES

SUGAR-FREE DESSERT SELECTIONS

It can be difficult to follow a diet for ulcerative colitis (UC), but there are ways to enjoy sweets without making symptoms worse. One way to sweeten desserts without making blood sugar spikes is to use natural sweeteners like stevia or monk fruit extract instead of refined sugar. Recipes also frequently call for almond or coconut flour instead of traditional flours because they are less carbohydrate-rich and easier on the stomach.

Avocado chocolate mousse, for example, combines ripe avocados with cocoa powder and a small amount of honey for sweetness. Its creamy texture provides healthy fats and antioxidants while satisfying cravings. Chia seed pudding, on the other hand, is made with chia seeds, unsweetened almond milk, and a dash of vanilla extract. Rich in fiber, chia seeds support digestive health and help stabilize blood sugar levels. These desserts are low-sugar and nutritious enough to support an ulcerative colitis management plan.

FRUIT-BASED SWEETS

Fruits are a great way to get natural sweetness and important nutrients into desserts. If you have ulcerative colitis, you should choose fruits that are easy to digest. Here are some simple but tasty ideas: grilling peaches with honey and cinnamon to caramelize the fruit's natural sugars and make it sweeter without adding extra sugar. Another idea is to make a mixed berry parfait with fresh berries, dairy-free yogurt, and granola for crunch and fiber.

Fruit sorbet is another option; it's made by blending frozen fruits like mangoes or berries with a little citrus juice. Sorbets are light and refreshing, and since they don't contain dairy, they're easy on the stomach.

Fruit-based treats also offer fiber, vitamins, and antioxidants that support gut health overall and satisfy cravings for dessert in a way that's UC-friendly.

NON-DAIRY ICE CREAMS

Dairy-free alternatives are better because they don't contain lactose or casein and have a creamy texture without causing problems for some people with ulcerative colitis.

Dairy-free ice creams are typically made with almond or coconut milk as the base and can be customized to taste better with fruits or natural sweeteners.

One recipe calls for combining full-fat coconut milk, vanilla extract, and a small amount of maple syrup with churning and freezing to make a velvety treat that can be flavored with chopped nuts or dairy-free chocolate chips. Another is banana ice cream, which is made by freezing ripe bananas and pureeing them until smooth. The natural sweetness and creamy texture of the bananas make for a simple, satisfying dessert that's easy on the stomach.

GUT-RELEASING GELATIN TREATS

Fruit gelatin cups combine gelatin powder with fruit juice or herbal tea for a light and refreshing dessert option. These cups are easy to digest and can be made with low-sugar or natural sweeteners to suit dietary preferences. Gelatin desserts can be soothing for the gut due to their gentle properties and potential to support digestive health. Gelatin is derived from animal collagen and is known for its ability to promote gut integrity and ease inflammation.

Collagen protein bites, which combine gelatin powder, nut butter, coconut flakes, and honey, are an additional suggestion. Packed with protein and healthy fats, these bites make a filling snack or dessert. Gelatin desserts are a treat for the palate as well as a good addition to a UC-friendly diet because they support gut health.

UC-FRIENDLY PASTRIES

Eating baked goods while managing ulcerative colitis means choosing ingredients that are easy on the stomach. Recipes frequently call for alternative flours, such as oat flour or almond flour, which are easier to digest and lower in gluten. For example, ripe bananas combined with oat flour, eggs, and a little honey make for moist and flavorful muffins that make a healthy snack or dessert.

Almond flour cookies provide a nutty flavor and a dose of healthy fats; dark chocolate adds antioxidants without being overly sweet; these baked goods can be enjoyed in moderation as part of a balanced diet for managing ulcerative colitis, offering both nutritional value and satisfaction. Another idea is to make almond flour cookies with coconut oil, a natural sweetener such as maple syrup, and dark chocolate chips.

DRINKS AND SMOOTHIES

DRINKS THAT REHYDRATE FOR UC

Maintaining proper hydration is essential for the management of ulcerative colitis (UC), as dehydration can worsen symptoms. Hydrating beverages should concentrate on restoring fluids without upsetting the digestive system. Basic choices include plain water flavored with a squeeze of citrus, which hydrates without adding sugars or artificial ingredients that may aggravate symptoms. Another great option is coconut water, which is rich in electrolytes, such as potassium and magnesium, which support hydration and muscle function. It is also easy on the stomach and can be calming during flare-ups.

In addition to providing hydration and calming effects, herbal teas like ginger tea or chamomile steep in hot water for several minutes, strain, and drink. Teas high in tannins or caffeine can be harsh on the lining of the stomach.

Herbal teas are also known for their anti-inflammatory qualities, which can help reduce inflammation in the gut.

Slicing fruits like cucumbers or berries into infused water is a tasty way to add some natural sweetness and antioxidants that support gut health in general. Some UC patients may be able to handle diluted fruit juices but be sure to choose low-acid varieties and dilute them with water to lessen their acidity. In the end, UC patients should stick to simple drinks that don't contain too much sugar, acid, or artificial additives that could aggravate their symptoms.

TEAS WITH ANTI-INFLAMMATION

By reducing inflammation in the digestive tract, anti-inflammatory teas can be extremely helpful in the management of ulcerative colitis. One popular anti-inflammatory tea is ginger tea, which can help reduce symptoms such as bloating and abdominal pain. It is made by steeping fresh ginger slices in hot water for a few minutes, straining, and then drinking.

Honey, which also has antibacterial properties, can be added for sweetness.

Due to the active compound in turmeric, curcumin, this spice has been shown in studies to help reduce inflammation in conditions similar to ulcerative cystitis. To make turmeric tea, add ground turmeric to hot water along with a pinch of black pepper (which helps absorb curcumin) and simmer for a few minutes before straining. You can also add a dash of cinnamon or a squeeze of lemon to enhance the earthy flavor of the tea.

Herbal blends containing licorice root or peppermint can also be beneficial, as they aid in digestion and provide additional anti-inflammatory benefits. Because chamomile tea is so well-known for its calming properties, it can help reduce the discomfort and spasms associated with ulcerative cystitis (UC). When selecting anti-inflammatory teas for UC, go for organic varieties to reduce exposure to pesticides and other potential irritants.

SMOOTHIES PACKED WITH NUTRIENTS

Smoothies that are loaded with nutrients are a quick and easy way to support gut health, especially when there are flare-ups or periods of low appetite. Begin with a base of easily digested liquids, such as coconut water or almond milk, which provide electrolytes and hydration; add fruits, such as bananas, which are easy on the stomach and provide potassium to regulate muscle function and fluid balance; and finish with antioxidant-rich berries, which have anti-inflammatory qualities.

Add leafy greens, like spinach or kale, to increase nutritional content. These high-fiber, vitamin- and mineral-rich foods support digestive health in general and can help regulate bowel movements. Add a scoop of plain yogurt or a plant-based protein powder that is free of additives and artificial sweeteners. Add some healthy fats and fiber, like flaxseeds or chia seeds, to aid in digestion and provide a feeling of fullness.

Nutrient-packed smoothies not only provide vital vitamins and minerals but also help maintain energy levels and promote healing during periods of gastrointestinal distress. Blend well to ensure easy digestion. Avoid ingredients known to trigger symptoms, such as high-acid fruits or excessive amounts of fiber. Experiment with different combinations to find what works best for your individual needs and tolerances.

MAKE YOUR ELECTROLYTE DRINKS

In contrast to commercial sports drinks that frequently contain high levels of sugar and artificial additives, homemade versions of electrolyte drinks can be tailored to provide hydration without exacerbating symptoms, which is important for individuals with UC, especially during flare-ups when dehydration is a concern. To begin, start with a base of coconut water, which naturally contains electrolytes like potassium and magnesium, crucial for maintaining fluid balance and muscle function.

For an added taste and nutritional boost, try adding a pinch of sea salt (sodium is another important electrolyte that helps the body regulate water levels) to your drink instead of table salt (which may contain additives that irritate the digestive tract). Freshly squeezed citrus juice (vitamin C and antioxidants that support immune function and gut health) also adds flavor.

Make your electrolyte drink by experimenting with different combinations of ingredients to find a drink that tastes good and meets your hydration needs during periods of UC flare-ups.

Herbs like mint or basil also add refreshing flavors without irritating the stomach; for sweetness, use stevia or honey sparingly, though it's best to limit added sugars to avoid potential triggers.

DRINKING AND UC: THINGS TO CONSIDER

Alcohol can irritate the lining of the digestive tract and exacerbate inflammation, making it a potential trigger for flare-ups in individuals with ulcerative colitis (UC). It is important to approach alcohol consumption cautiously and consider its impact on your specific symptoms and overall well-being. A comprehensive understanding of the relationship between alcohol consumption and ulcerative colitis is essential for managing symptoms and overall health.

Since alcohol can upset the balance of gut bacteria and interfere with medications prescribed to manage symptoms, it is generally advised that people with UC limit or avoid alcohol completely, especially during flare-ups or when symptoms are active. Certain beverages, like wine and beer, contain compounds like histamine and sulfites that can cause gastrointestinal symptoms and inflammation in sensitive people.

Always check with your healthcare provider about whether alcohol consumption is safe for you and how it may interact with your UC management plan. If you choose to drink, do so in moderation and pay attention to how your body responds.

CHAPTER SEVEN

FREQUENTLY ASKED QUESTIONS

HANDLING RELAPSES AND DIETARY MODIFICATIONS

Managing your diet is essential during ulcerative colitis (UC) flare-ups to reduce symptoms and facilitate healing. To start, stick to a low-residue diet to minimize fiber intake and facilitate digestion. This means avoiding raw fruits and vegetables, whole grains, nuts, and seeds; instead, choose well-cooked, peeled, or canned varieties. Lean meats, eggs, and fish are your best bet for easily digested protcins. Finally, introduce small, frequent meals to minimize stress on the digestive system.

A dietitian with expertise in UC can offer customized advice for successful flare management through dietary modifications. Restrictions may include cutting out trigger foods that worsen symptoms, such as dairy, spicy foods, and high-fat items; maintaining a food diary to track reactions and identify personal triggers;

gradually reintroducing foods after a flare under supervision to assess tolerance levels; and making sure you're properly hydrated with water and electrolytes to support digestion and prevent dehydration during episodes.

HANDLING MALNUTRITION AND WEIGHT LOSS

Malnutrition and weight loss are common concerns for people with UC, particularly during flare-ups. To effectively manage weight loss, concentrate on foods that are high in nutrients and easy on the digestive tract. Include small, frequent meals that are high in calories and protein to sustain muscle mass and energy levels. Nutrient-dense foods include white rice, bananas, cooked vegetables without skins, and smooth nut butter.

To prevent malnutrition, make sure that all nutrients are absorbed even in the case of dietary restrictions. If eating solid foods is difficult, think about using protein powders or liquid supplements to increase caloric intake. Regularly check vitamin and mineral levels because malabsorption can lead to deficiencies.

Consult a healthcare professional to determine the right amount of supplements to take based on your specific needs and symptoms. These tactics can help control weight loss and preserve overall nutritional balance when UC activity is occurring.

UC TRAVELING AND DINING OUT

For people with UC, traveling and eating out can be difficult, but with careful planning, these situations can be managed well. Before you travel, research potential destinations and restaurants that serve food that fits into a UC-friendly diet. Look for places that offer simple preparations like steamed vegetables and grilled proteins, or that offer customizable dishes. Bring along portable snacks like rice cakes, nut butter, or low-fiber crackers to have on hand in case your options for suitable food are limited.

When traveling, stay hydrated to support digestive health and prevent dehydration. Carry emergency supplies and medications in case of unexpected flare-ups.

By planning and making informed choices, people with UC can enjoy travel and dining experiences while effectively managing their dietary needs. Communicate your dietary needs to restaurant staff so that meals are prepared according to your preferences and restrictions.

FOOD ALLERGIES AND SENSITIVITIES

Managing food sensitivities and allergies is crucial for individuals with UC to prevent flare-ups and discomfort. Identify trigger foods through an elimination diet or allergy testing to pinpoint specific allergens or intolerances. Common triggers include gluten, dairy, artificial sweeteners, and certain preservatives. Once identified, eliminate trigger foods from your diet to alleviate symptoms and promote digestive comfort.

Read food labels carefully to avoid hidden allergens and cross-contamination risks. Substitute triggers ingredients with suitable alternatives to maintain a balanced diet without compromising nutritional needs. Consider working with a registered dietitian to create a personalized meal plan that accommodates specific food sensitivities while ensuring adequate nutrient intake. By proactively managing food sensitivities and allergies, individuals with UC can optimize digestive health and minimize the risk of symptom flare-ups.

LONG-TERM DIETARY MANAGEMENT STRATEGIES

Long-term dietary management for ulcerative colitis involves establishing sustainable eating habits that support gut health and overall well-being. Adopt a balanced diet rich in lean proteins, fruits, and vegetables while moderating intake of high-fat, spicy, and processed foods known to exacerbate symptoms. Incorporate probiotics-rich foods like yogurt or kefir to promote a healthy gut microbiome and aid indigestion.

Following these guidelines can help individuals with UC achieve sustained symptom relief and improve their quality of life through effective dietary choices. Gradually implementing dietary modifications facilitates better adaptation and symptom management.

Regularly monitoring symptoms and dietary responses can help identify patterns and make necessary adjustments. Physical activity regularly supports digestive function and overall health. Seek ongoing guidance from healthcare providers and dietitians specializing in gastrointestinal health to optimize long-term dietary management strategies tailored to individual needs.

www.ingramcontent.com/pod-product-compliance
Lightning Source LLC
Chambersburg PA
CBHW071837210526
45479CB00001B/171